VEGAN ABCs

Written by Debra J. Mines

Photography by Asante M. Fears

Kindle Direct Publishing
https://kdp.amazon.com

Table of Contents

Foreword

The author, Debra J. Mines, wrote **VEGAN ABCs** to provide an enjoyable strategy for moms to teach their young children to appreciate fruits and vegetables while learning to read the alphabet in English and to connect the letters to non-fiction, true-to-life vegan foods.

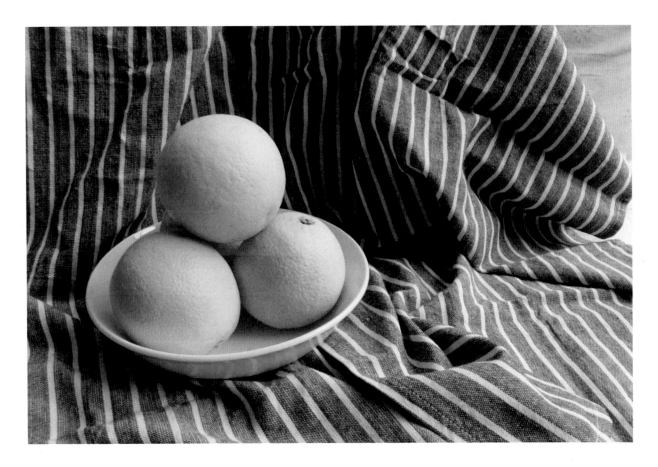

Debra J. Mines writes books to teach children how to read and to become fluent readers.

Since she wrote **VEGAN ABCs** for beginning readers, she has provided large, distinguishable upper-case and lower-case letters with clcar, captivating pictures to match the letters. She also included practice and research activities at the end of the book.

Enjoy Reading!

Dedication

This book is dedicated to my children, Hermalena V. Mines Powell and Clifford H. Mines; my son-in-law, Matthew A. Powell; and my grandchildren, Alaina and Alan Powell, who are eating more vegetables and fruits today than they did yesterday.

Special Thanks

Alton Delmore, my cousin, receives special thanks for encouraging me to continue to write books for young children and for children of all ages.

Steve Won receives special thanks for sparking my interest in writing **VEGAN ABCs** as a non-fiction alternative to the book, **STINKY ABCs**, which I wrote and published in 2022.

Special notes of thanks also are given to Dr. Carol Kellyman, Beverly London, and Tonya Washington for offering the names of various fruits and vegetables to include in **VEGAN ABCs** and/or for suggesting places to shop for food items such as the ones that begin with the letters "U, X, Y, and Z".

Special thanks are given to Andrew and Maricel Powell for assisting with the pronunciation of Ube (oo- bay or oo-beh), a purple yam.

Finally, special thanks are given to Szuchi Young for assisting with the pronunciation of Xing (shing), a Chinese apricot.

All friends and relatives identified above helped to make the writing of **VEGAN ABCs** a unique and worthwhile experience.

FRUIT or VEGETABLE?

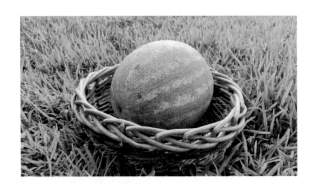
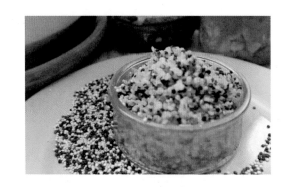
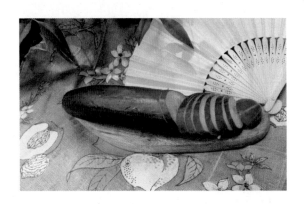
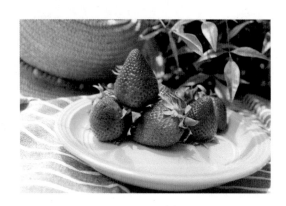
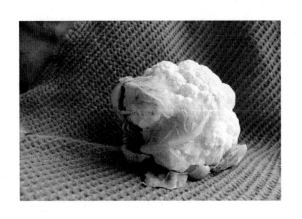
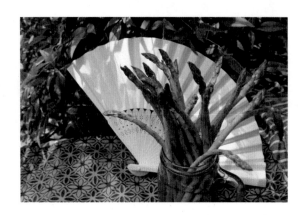

1

Aa
is for asparagus.

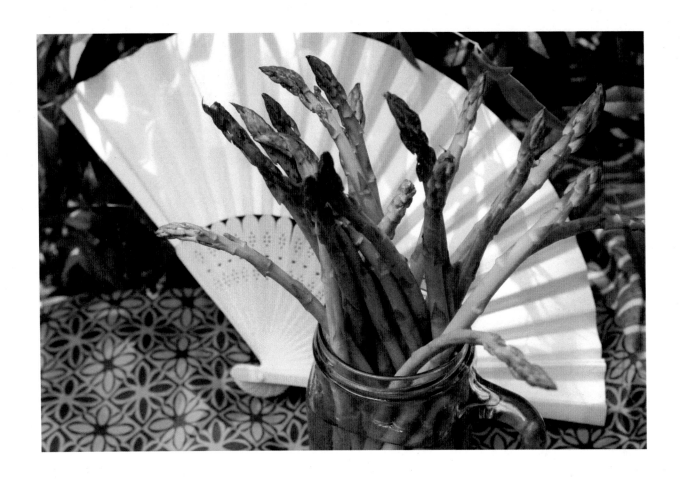

Bb
is for banana.

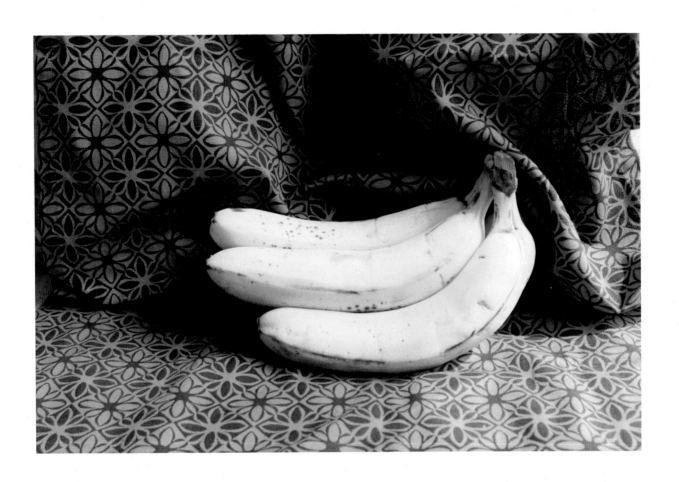

Cc
is for cauliflower.

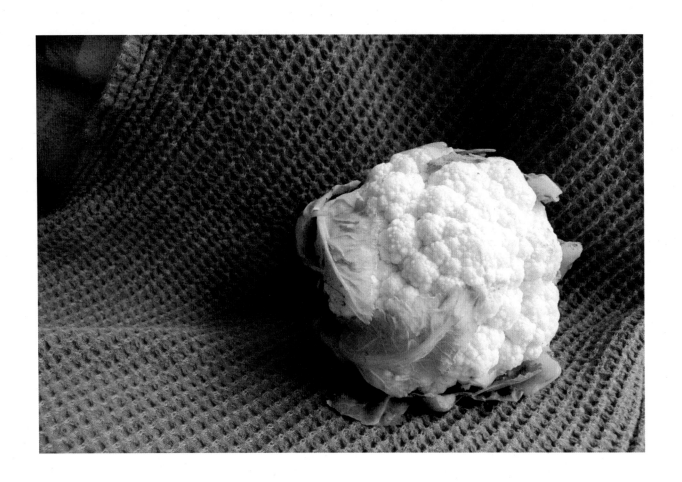

Dd
is for dill.

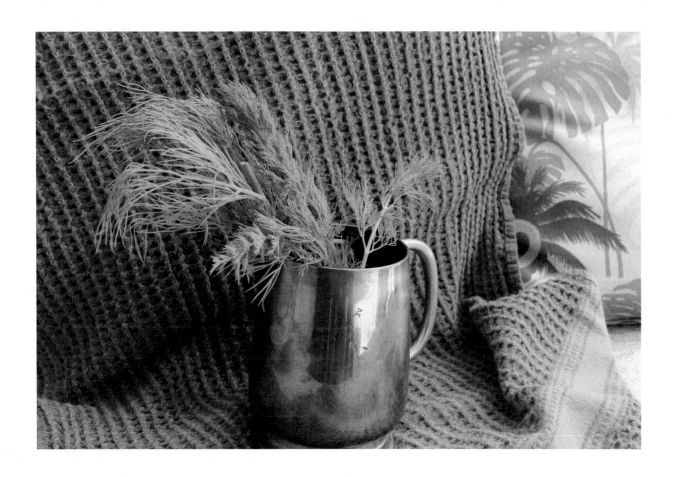

Ee
is for edamame.

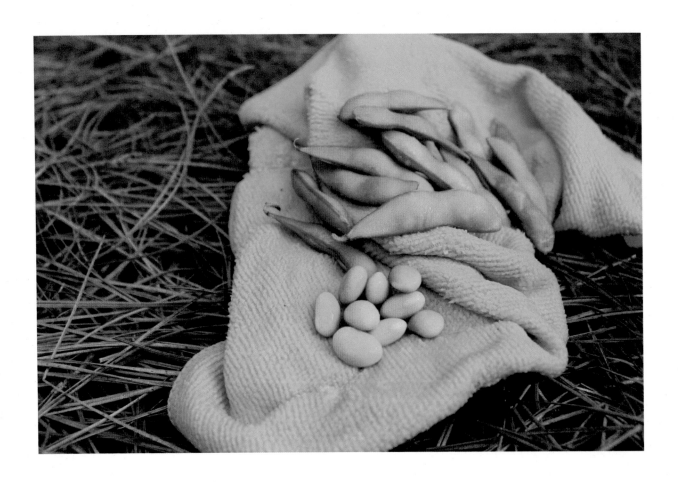

Ff
is for fennel.

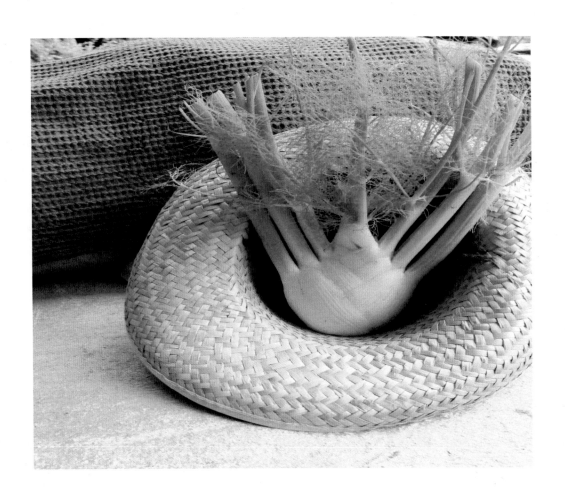

Gg
is for garlic.

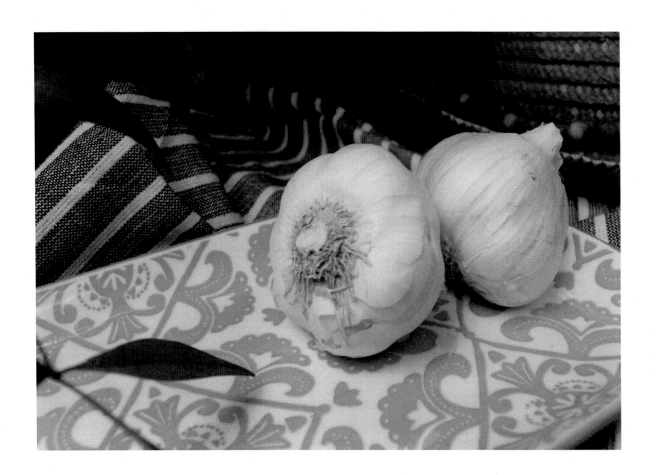

Hh

is for hot peppers.

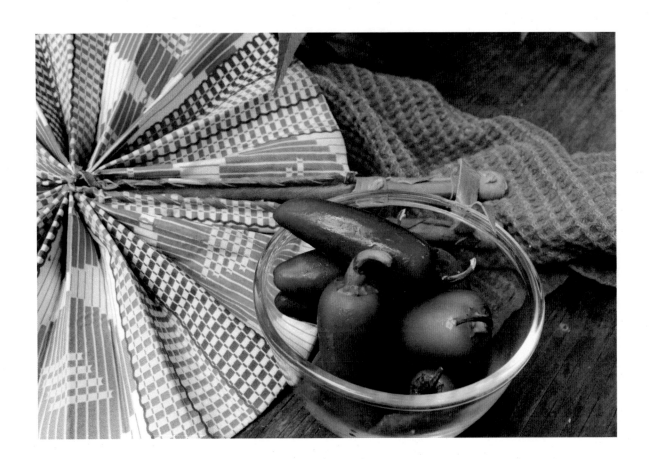

Ii

is for Indian Eggplants.

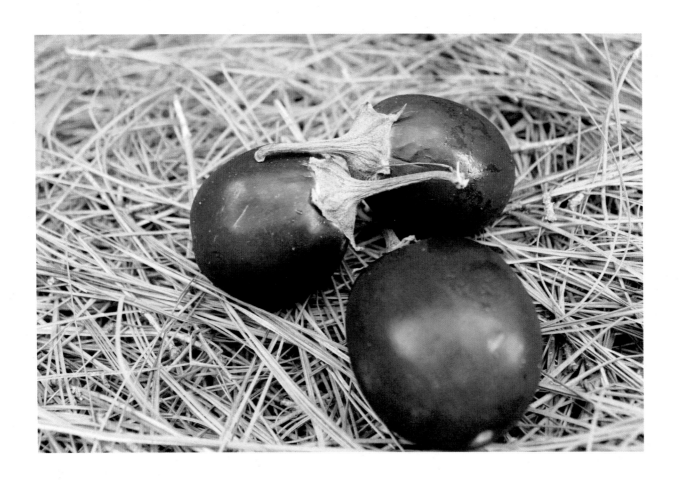

Jj
is for jackfruit.

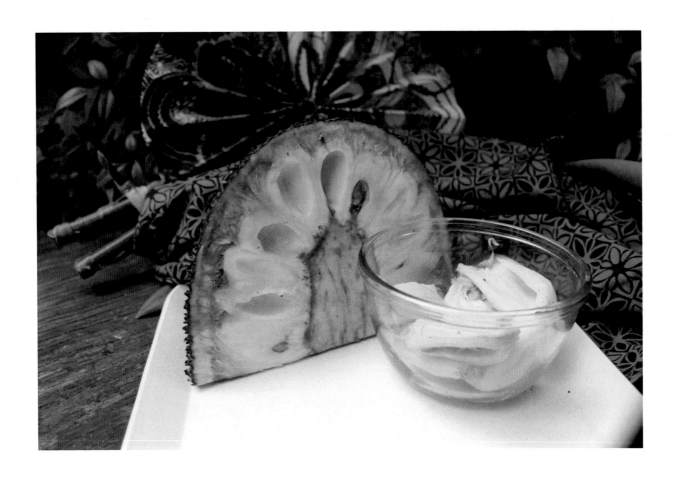

Kk
is for kiwi.

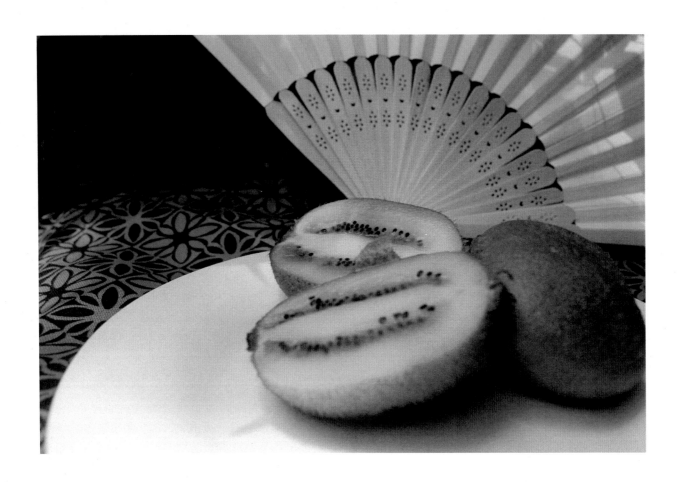

Ll
is for lemon.

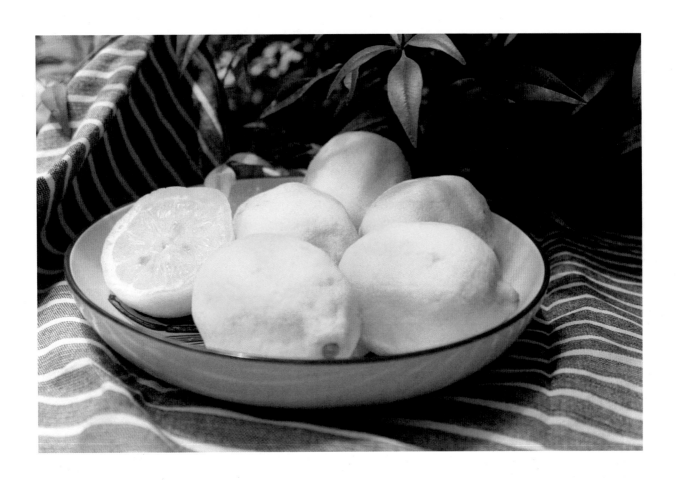

Mm
is for mushrooms.

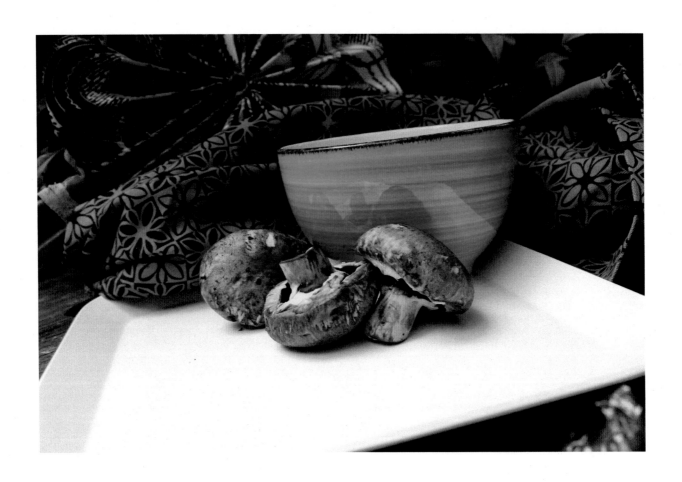

Nn
is for nectarines.

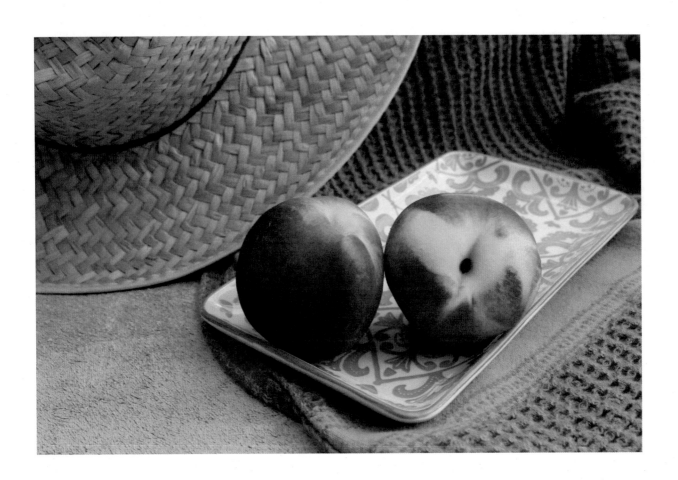

Oo
is for okra.

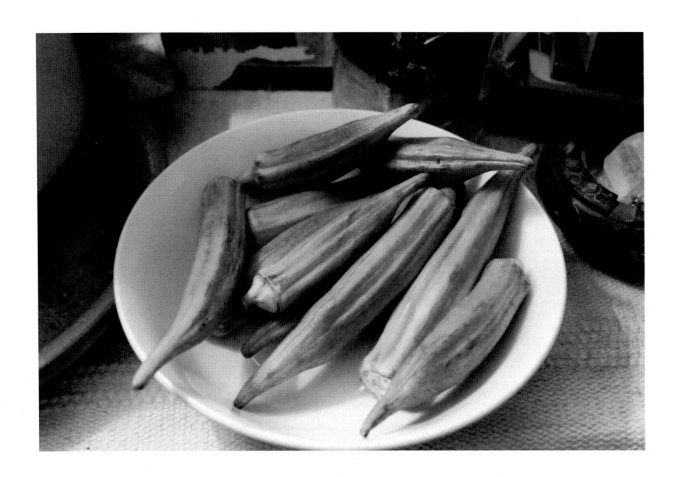

Pp
is for pineapple.

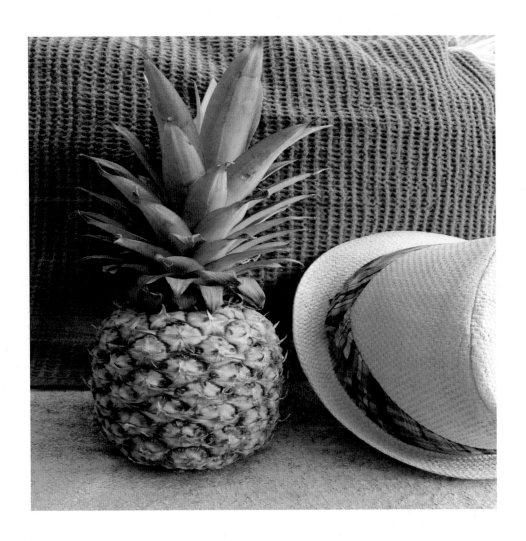

Qq
is for quinoa.

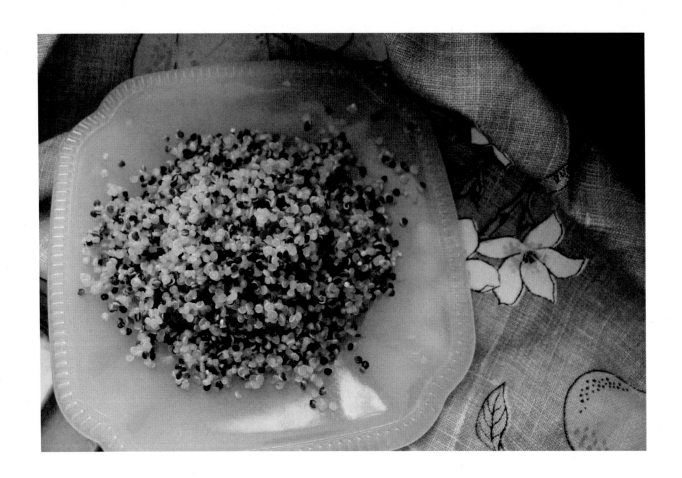

Rr
is for Red Cabbage.

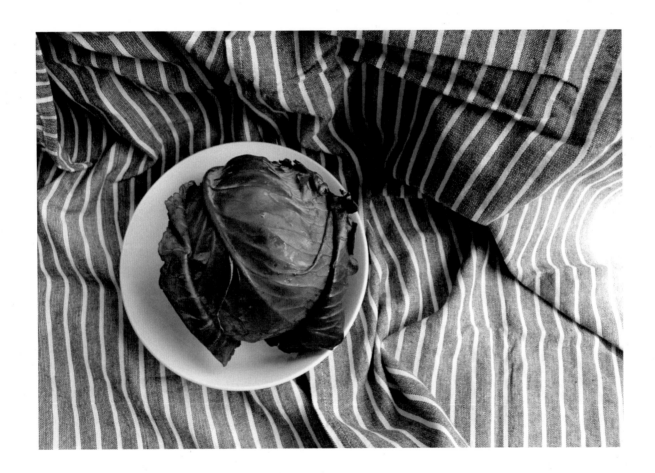

Ss
is for strawberries.

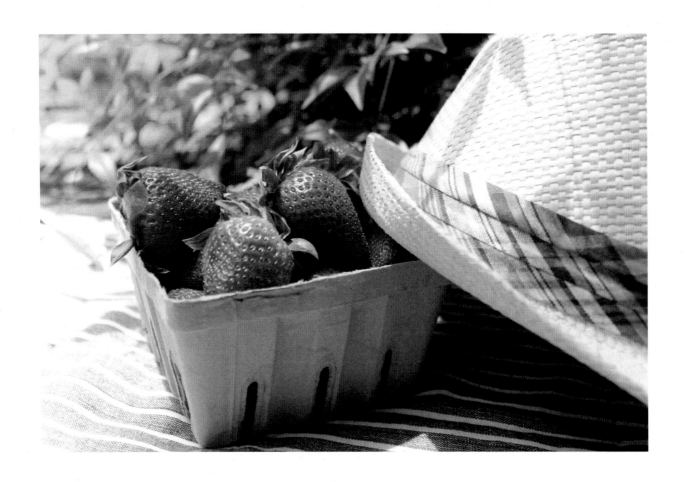

Tt
is for turmeric.

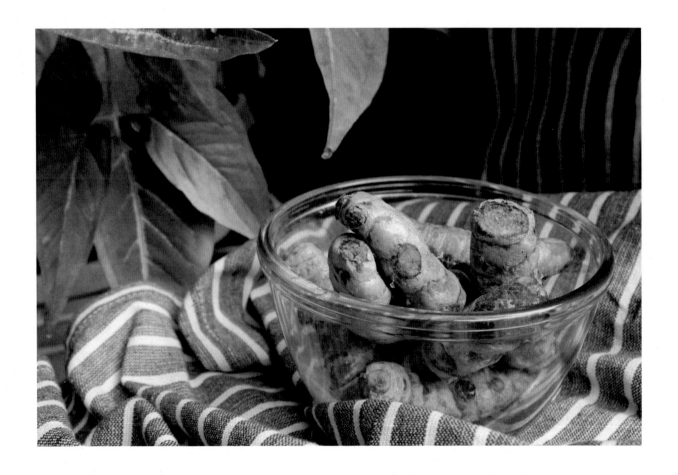

Uu

is for ube (OO-bay or OO-beh,

a purple yam).

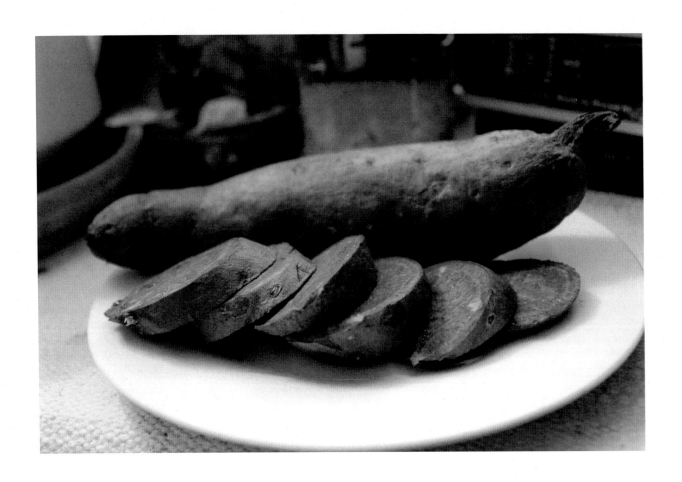

Vv
is for Valencia Oranges.

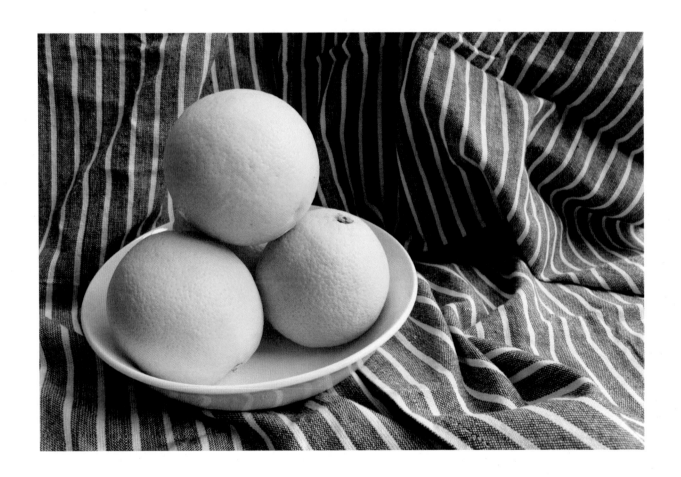

Ww
is for watermelon.

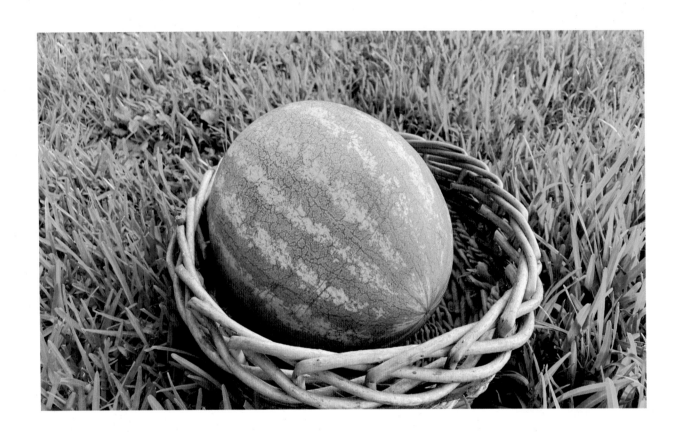

24

Xx

is for xing (shing,

a Chinese apricot).

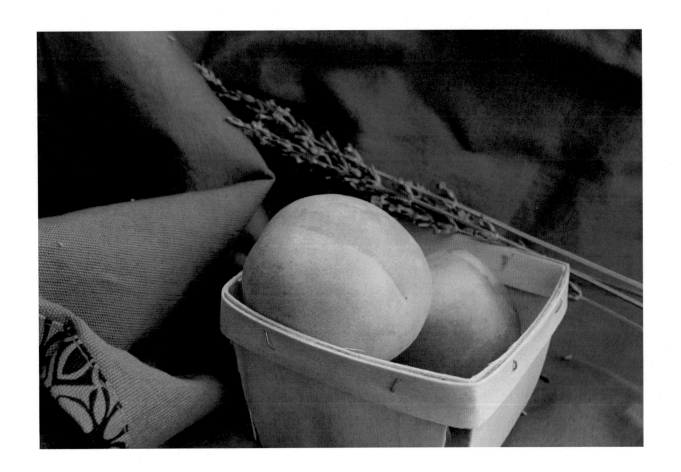

Yy
is for Yellow Dragon Fruit.

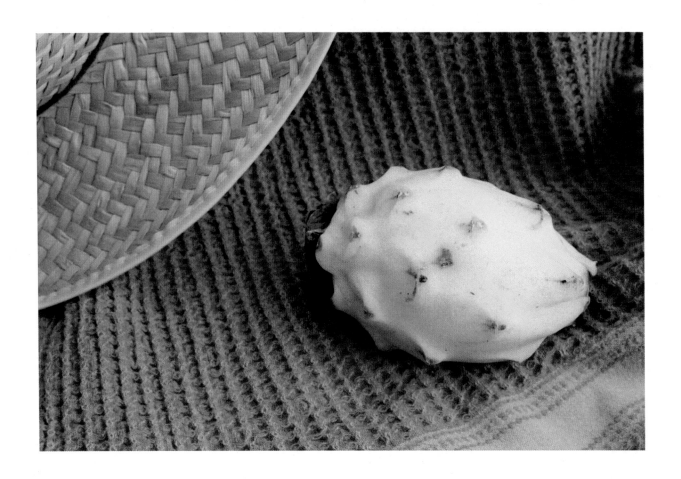

Zz
is for zucchini.

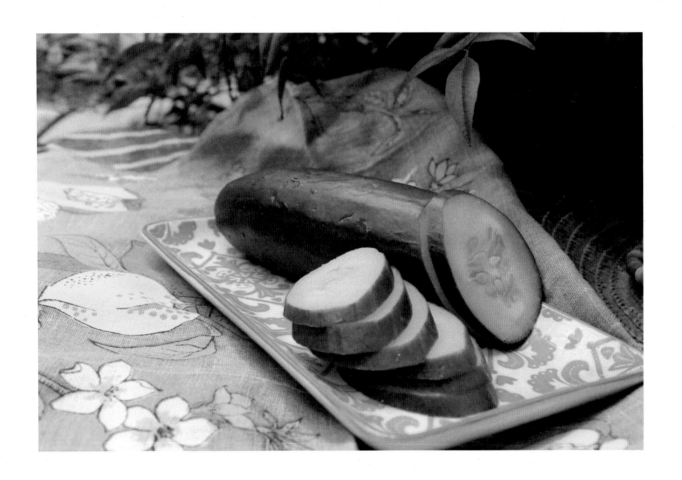

DIRECTIONS for ACTIVITY 1

1. Look at the word bank on page 29.
2. Choose words from the word bank to fill in the blank lines for each letter of the alphabet on pages 30 – 55.
3. Draw a picture for each letter of the alphabet on pages 30 - 55.

WORD BANK for ACTIVITY 1

zucchini	Yellow Dragon Fruit
asparagus	lemon
watermelon	ube (OO-bay or OO-beh)
banana	Valencia Oranges
turmeric	cauliflower
dill	strawberries
edamame	Red Cabbage
quinoa	Indian Eggplants
garlic	mushrooms
fennel	pineapple
okra	nectarines
kiwi	hot peppers
xing (shing)	jackfruit

Activity 1

Aa

_____.

Picture Box

Bb

_____.

Picture Box

31

Cc

_____.

Picture Box

32

Dd

_____.

Picture Box

33

Ee

_____.

Picture Box

34

Ff

_____.

Picture Box

35

Gg

_____.

Picture Box

Hh

_____.

```
┌─────────────────────────────────┐
│          Picture Box            │
│                                 │
│                                 │
│                                 │
│                                 │
│                                 │
│                                 │
│                                 │
│                                 │
│                                 │
│                                 │
│                                 │
└─────────────────────────────────┘
```

37

Ii

_____.

Picture Box

Jj

_____.

Picture Box

Kk

_____.

```
┌─────────────────────────────┐
│        Picture Box          │
│                             │
│                             │
│                             │
│                             │
│                             │
│                             │
│                             │
│                             │
│                             │
│                             │
└─────────────────────────────┘
```

Ll

_____.

```
┌─────────────────────────────────┐
│          Picture Box            │
│                                 │
│                                 │
│                                 │
│                                 │
│                                 │
│                                 │
│                                 │
│                                 │
│                                 │
│                                 │
│                                 │
│                                 │
└─────────────────────────────────┘
```

41

Mm

_____ .

```
┌─────────────────────────────────────┐
│            Picture Box                │
│                                       │
│                                       │
│                                       │
│                                       │
│                                       │
│                                       │
│                                       │
│                                       │
│                                       │
│                                       │
└─────────────────────────────────────┘
```

42

Nn

_____.

Picture Box

Oo

_____.

```
┌─────────────────────────────────┐
│          Picture Box            │
│                                 │
│                                 │
│                                 │
│                                 │
│                                 │
│                                 │
│                                 │
│                                 │
│                                 │
│                                 │
│                                 │
└─────────────────────────────────┘
```

44

Pp

_____.

Picture Box

45

Qq

_____.

Picture Box

46

Rr

_____.

Picture Box

47

Ss

_____.

Picture Box

48

Tt

_____.

Picture Box

49

Uu

_____.

+-------------------------------+
| Picture Box |
| |
| |
| |
| |
| |
| |
| |
| |
+-------------------------------+

Vv

_____.

Picture Box

Ww

_____ .

```
┌─────────────────────────────────────┐
│              Picture Box              │
│                                       │
│                                       │
│                                       │
│                                       │
│                                       │
│                                       │
│                                       │
│                                       │
│                                       │
│                                       │
│                                       │
│                                       │
│                                       │
└─────────────────────────────────────┘
```

Xx

_____.

Picture Box

53

Yy

_____.

Picture Box

Zz

_____.

Picture Box

55

Answer Key for Activity 1

Aa   is for asparagus.

Bb   is for banana.

Cc   is for cauliflower.

Dd   is for dill.

Ee   is for edamame.

Ff   is for fennel.

Gg   is for garlic.

Hh   is for hot peppers.

Ii   is for Indian Eggplants.

Jj   is for jackfruit.

Kk   is for kiwi.

Ll   is for lemon.

Mm   is for mushrooms.

Nn   is for nectarines.

Oo   is for okra.

Pp   is for pineapple.

Qq   is for quinoa.

Rr   is for Red Cabbage.

Ss   is for strawberries.

Tt   is for turmeric.

Uu   is for ube.

Vv   is for Valencia Oranges.

Ww   is for watermelon.

Xx   is for xing.

Yy   is for Yellow Dragon Fruit.

Zz   is for zucchini.

Activity 2

Can you read the book, <u>Vegan ABCs</u>, again and write answers on the blank lines below?

Aa is for _____.

Bb is for _____.

Cc is for _____.

Dd is for _____.

Ee is for _____.

Ff is for _____.

Gg is for _____.

Hh is for _____.

Ii is for _____.

Jj is for _____.

Kk is for _____.

Ll is for _____.

Mm is for _____.

Nn is for _____.

Oo is for _____.

Pp is for _____.

Qq is for _____.

Rr is for _____.

Ss is for _____.

Tt is for _____.

Uu is for _____.

Vv is for _____.

Ww is for _____.

Xx is for _____.

Yy is for _____.

Zz is for _____.

Answer Key for Activity 2

Aa   is for asparagus.

Bb   is for banana.

Cc   is for cauliflower.

Dd   is for dill.

Ee   is for edamame.

Ff   is for fennel.

Gg   is for garlic.

Hh   is for hot peppers.

Ii   is for Indian Eggplants.

Jj   is for jackfruit.

Kk   is for kiwi.

Ll   is for lemon.

Mm is for mushrooms.

Nn   is for nectarines.

Oo   is for okra.

Pp   is for pineapple.

Qq   is for quinoa.

Rr   is for Red Cabbage.

Ss   is for strawberries.

Tt   is for turmeric.

Uu   is for ube.

Vv   is for Valencia Oranges.

Ww   is for watermelon.

Xx   is for xing.

Yy   is for Yellow Dragon Fruit.

Zz   is for zucchini.

RESEARCH PROJECT 1

1. What is your favorite fruit?

   _____.

2. Draw a picture of your favorite fruit.

RESEARCH PROJECT 1
continued

3. Where does your fruit grow? What is your fruit's origin?

_____

_____.

4. Describe the seeds in your favorite fruit.

_____

_____.

5. Write one or two sentences about your favorite fruit.

_____

_____

_____

_____.

RESEARCH PROJECT 2

1. What is your favorite vegetable?

_____.

2. Draw a picture of your favorite vegetable.

RESEARCH PROJECT 2
continued

3. Where does your vegetable grow? What is your vegetable's

    origin? _____

    _____.

4. Does your vegetable plant have leaves, a stalk, roots, tubers,
    bulbs, or flowers?

    _____

    _____.

5. How does your vegetable taste?

    _____

    _____.

6. Write one sentence about your favorite vegetable.

    _____

    _____.

About the Author

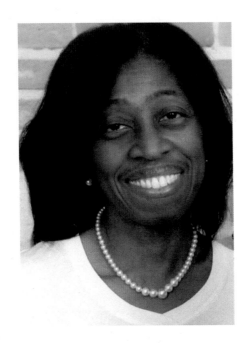

Debra J. (Thomas) Mines grew up in Cleveland, Ohio, USA. After graduating from East High School, she attended Ohio Wesleyan University and graduated with a Bachelor of Arts Degree in Elementary Education with a concentration in Reading instruction. Soon after graduation, she married the late Herman C. Mines and enjoyed family life with him and their two children, whom they read to continuously. During these years she also graduated from Case Western Reserve University with a Master of Arts Degree in Curriculum and Instruction with a specialization in Reading Supervision. Additionally, she completed all but the dissertation for a doctorate in Educational Administration from the University of Akron and later achieved the distinction of being a National Board-Certified Teacher (NBCT).

Debra J. (Thomas) Mines has taught children to read and write from pre-school through twelfth grade. Additional highlights of her career include teaching graduate-level courses as a part-time instructor at Cleveland State University and teaching graduate courses for the Summer Institute for Reading Intervention sponsored by Ohio's Northeast Regional Professional Development Center.

About the Author continued:

As a professional teacher and life-long learner, Debra J. Mines is compelled to learn as much as possible about her students, their cultures, and their communities. This desire motivated her to complete programs for the English to Speakers of Other Languages (ESOL) Endorsement and the Gifted In-Field Endorsement. She enjoys teaching diverse populations of students and looks forward to continuing to share her stories, knowledge, and skills to help each child to reach his/her highest potential.

Vegan ABCs is the third book written by Debra J. Mines. Other books written by the author are *Stinky Shoes* and *Stinky ABCs*. Additional books are forthcoming. Enjoy reading each book!

Visit https://www.stinkyshoes.shop for more information.

About the Photographer

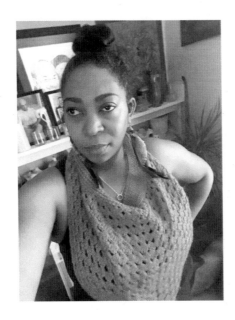

Artist, designer, and Photographer

Asante M. Fears is a self-taught Artist with minimal formal training. She studied for a few years at Georgia State University in Studio Art. She also has a B.S. in Marketing from Albany State University.

She enjoys doing volunteer work as an artist. She worked as Art Instructor for "ChopArt", a non-profit that allows homeless teens to express themselves constructively. She was involved in this for five years until 2020. She exhibited her works at many different spaces around the city of Atlanta. She belongs to an artist group by the name of "Sistagraphy", a group of women photographers.

She has enjoyed photographing since a young child. She believes that a photograph holds a precious memory locked forever. Her technique has been developed by trial and error. Once it was locked, she then decided on what she would focus on as far as her photography. As a photographer she enjoys Documentary Photography, lifestyle photography, and still life photography.